Yellow
Butterfly

Yellow Butterfly

Poetry, Art, and Photography

by

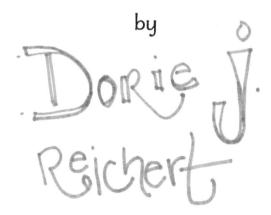

A creative talent's struggle with
mental illness.

Prepared by North Star Press of St. Cloud Inc.

www.northstarpress.com

ISBN: 978-1-68201-154-6

First Edition

Type set in Filson Pro Book and Charcuterie Flared.

All poems, prose, and interior artwork by Dorie Reichert.

Cover design and interior layout by Liz Dwyer of North Star Press.

Contents

Praise for *Yellow Butterfly*

Dorie Reichert's posthumous book of poetry, Yellow Butterfly, is a hauntingly beautiful and eloquent glimpse into the beginnings of what could have been, were not for an encounter with bipolar disorder. Through her poetry Reichert guides us along the path of her creative experience to a place where we can start to empathize with a "mind (that) has been split open too many times." The potential of her creative voice, easily seen in her earliest work, becomes even more apparent in her later poems. Like a shore bird's tracks in the sand, her sparse but keen use of language reveals an authenticity of style and a sense of how far she may have gone on her poetic journey. Confessional at times, Dorie Reichert does not use these revelations to shock us but to help us begin to unpack her experience. Knowing all too well how the world outside of her illness misconceives the landscape she navigated, her poetry offers us a way inside of it by using direct and honest imagery: "...I would have my mind/ be a sharpened lance/and not a soft bruised fruit/ decaying slowly/awash in an ocean of words..." The poetry of Yellow Butterfly and its engaging introduction, written by her father, Bob Reichert, afford us a meaningful starting point for a long overdue and serious conversation about mental health.

-Steve Therrien,
High School English Teacher

Acknowledgments

While in college Dorie's sister, Mary Reichert Sannerud, wrote a long paper reflecting on Dorie's life and death. Several excerpts from Mary's paper in the introduction add to an understanding of Dorie's life. Mary also had helpful comments on introduction drafts, and on proofs of this book.

I am deeply grateful for my friend Faris Keeling, retired psychiatrist, who provided valuable assistance in preparing the introduction. He helped add focus and organization through a review and extensive comment on several drafts. Faris also helped to assure mental health references are presented correctly.

Dorie's mother, Kitty Van Evera, had helpful comments on a review of early introduction drafts.

Myriam J. A. Chancy, a college English professor and accomplished author and speaker, reviewed the entire collection of Dorie's poetry and short prose. Her selection and organization of Dorie's most compelling writing is the main body of this book.

Jeff Frey and his business CLP digitized all of Dorie's art work that is included in the book.

A delightful experience has been getting to know and work with Curtis and Liz Dwyer and their business North Star Press. Their book publishing talent and experience was instrumental in bringing this book to life.

I have many thanks and gratitude to everyone for all the help provided in producing this book of Dorie's work.

-Bob Reichert

FORWARD

When Bob Reichert asked for my help creating a book of Dorie's work, I agreed because of our friendship. I didn't realize it would actually become a valuable and unique contribution to understanding and treating the most serious type of mental illness—that with recurrent or chronic psychosis.

"Psychosis" means losing touch with reality, and shows up in symptoms such as delusions (persistent beliefs which are clearly false to others); hallucinations (sensing things that are not actually present); and/or disorganized thinking (which prevents understanding and thinking clearly about what is actually happening). These symptoms improve or resolve when treatment with medication is successful.

Yellow Butterfly's Introduction examines one family's experience with their loved-one's psychotic illness. But it is not just about Dorie and her family. Unfortunately, it describes a journey traveled by many, many Dories and families. The lessons learned are clearly stated, and could significantly improve outcomes for many patients and families.

But such good outcomes require that the person with illness understands that early, continuous, persistent treatment is in their own best interest. The usual pattern—as in Dorie's case—is going off and on medication multiple times. Each time off medication allows the illness to return more severely, causing a downward spiral of worsening disease over time.

Dorie's illness started with discrete episodes of psychosis; once medication took effect, she would return to her normal self. But after several more episodes triggered in part by stopping medication, the illness became more continuous, and resistant to treatment; she never again fully returned to her normal self.

But—for multiple reasons—it is very difficult for a person with such illness to stay on medication continuously, even when doing well. We need tools which increase understanding and motivation to take medication continuously.

Which is why Dorie's poems and illustrations are important. People with illness may or may not see themselves in the Introduction. But some will certainly recognize their own experience in Dorie's poems. Her poetry can help a person with illness better understand their inner experience during and between episodes of psychosis. Her poems also provide a cautionary tale, expressing her inner experience of disease progression— which might have been avoided by early and continuous treatment.

Faris Keeling MD
Psychiatrist (Retired)
Duluth, MN
March, 2023

INTRODUCTION

Dorie Reichert was a uniquely talented writer and visual artist, whose life and work would be compelling even without their insights into serious mental illness. She was—by her own description—an "unordinary" youth whose commitment to community service set an example for others regardless of age. "I'm not on a mission to solve all the world's problems, only to understand them." She recorded this mission in poetry, prose, drawings and photographs. They continue to challenge us to be true to our selves, and dare to see differently.

She was also my daughter.

Her life story- her youth and creative work prior to developing bipolar disorder, her clear expression of her experience with it, our family's struggle to get adequate treatment and engage her cooperation, the struggle to balance realistic coping and leading a normal life, and how the illness changed her—offers a cautionary tale. Here are clear lessons for people with serious mental illness, their loved ones, their mental health providers, and to all of us who need to better understand mental illness.

In addition, this book honors her request—made just days prior to her death—that her writings survive her. Here are some of her best poems, along with prose, drawings, and photographs. This introduction will present key points of her life story so that you can better understand the work of this "yellow butterfly" whose wings were clipped—perhaps unnecessarily- by serious mental illness.

HIGH SCHOOL,
& Her First Episode of Bipolar Illness

Dorie's years growing up were good ones. She felt supported in developing her intellectual curiosity, artistic talents and writing skills. She acquired a moral ethic of caring about and for others and for the environment.

From an autobiography for Dorie's ninth grade English class:

"...agates fascinate me. I love burning candles in my room. Stereo equipment is something I couldn't live without. I think that the music of Elvis Presley is revolting. I like broccoli. I believe that war is savage and proves nothing nor helps solve matters, only makes them worse. I think that watching television is a blatant waste of time and does nothing for expanding the powers of the mind, although it is relaxing. The rate at which our planet is deteriorating scares me. Teen magazines make me want to barf. I am not afraid of insects unless they are crawling or writhing on me. I dislike floral print bathroom wallpaper. I try the best I can to be sensitive to other people's needs. Moldy food turns me off. I sun burn easily. Poetry enthralls me. I wear M.C. Escher socks. I am not on a mission to solve all the world's problems, only to understand them. I do not wish to wear

braces. Child birth frightens me. I like Trident gum. I am unordinary."

She was also a normal child who enjoyed having fun and good times with friends. Dorie's sister, Mary, wrote:

"She spent her adolescent years in constant motion: asking questions, challenging rules, listening to Led Zeppelin and Pink Floyd loud, taking the car for joy rides, smoking on the front porch of the house, and having parties while our parents were away, all before she got her license.

"As Dorie grew older, her youthful energy was directed into what my parents thought were far more successful endeavors. She organized recycling programs and Earth Day events, ran the school greens club and edited the literary magazine, she worked at Play-Fair Discovery Center with youth on conflict resolution, and her senior year she won the Faculty Award."

Classmate Joel Kilgour writes about Dorie's volunteer work at Hannah House, a Catholic Worker homeless shelter in Duluth.

"I credit Dorie with being a major influence in my falling into the Catholic Worker movement. While we were still in high school, Dorie began volunteering for regular house shifts at Hannah House. She took on tasks most teenagers would shy away from—tending to daily chores and crisis calls, and caring for broken families. She was a thoughtful and hands-to-the-plow radical—running the school recycling program, volunteering her time at the house, or raising money for good causes."

3

Despite receiving the Duluth Marshall School's Faculty Award, the highest award given to a graduating senior, the end of her senior year in 1995 was difficult. As sometimes happens at that age she started experiencing symptoms which marked the onset of Bipolar Disorder. She struggled with the developing illness for a while until a high school counselor convinced her of the need to be hospitalized which lasted a full week. Yet, like many teens, she refused to take medication for her illness and as a result continued to struggle with the illness. So she suffered through it until mid-summer when she agreed to start taking medication. Soon she was back to the Dorie I knew before the illness started.

COLLEGE and PSYCHOSIS

4

Dorie was attracted to Warren Wilson College in Asheville, North Carolina because it emphasized the environment and required that students work an on-campus job and perform community service. Her two years there were a good, productive and happy time for Dorie. Even so, she must have had some mental health struggles since the first poem in this book about Manic Depression (Page 23) was written during her second year at Warren Wilson. **Those years were the last extended happy time in her life.** Too much of her life from then on was consumed by mental illness.

For her third year she transferred to Macalester College in Saint Paul, Minnesota. That year went well until the spring semester in 1998 when her mental illness returned with a vengeance. This time her manic depressive illness was complicated by psychosis, and police intervention was required to take her to a hospital in Saint Paul, kicking and screaming the whole way.

After several days in the hospital in Saint Paul she transferred to a Duluth hospital to be closer to home. The psychiatrist in Duluth recommended a commitment hearing because she believed that Dorie needed to be in the hospital for a longer period of time to stabilize her illness. However, at the hearing the psychiatrist did not make this clear to the judge, so Dorie was discharged. I had no choice but to take a very ill Dorie to our home in a situation of a relative new marriage for me and my wife. That was exceedingly stressful for all of us and the next few months were difficult.

Dorie slowly improved, but she never fully recovered.

RETURN to COLLEGE and a RETURN to PSYCHOSIS

After several months she felt ready to return to college. But rather than return to Macalester, she decided to attend Evergreen College in Olympia Washington, which has a strong, environmental emphasis and where students could design their own path of study. I did not want her to go far from home when not fully well, but in December 1998 she moved to Olympia to continue her college education.

She initially shared housing with several other women students, but had a hard time getting along with them. Her mental health gradually went downhill. In August, 1999 she wrote:

> *"Not too many things keeping me in check right now. Feeling myself beyond limits, group community knits me together a bit but makes me feel apart."*

So, that fall she moved into a trailer home. By then her sister, Mary, had moved to Portland Oregon. I was glad to have her near Dorie, and they enjoyed visiting with each other in Olympia and Portland.

Mary alerted us to problems as the next episode was building, but there was little we could do about it. She later wrote about one afternoon in late winter 2000:

> *"We were talking on the phone making plans to meet in Portland, and I began to recognize a distant, paranoid voice within my sister. She was talking fast. She was worried about her friend Ruth, who lived in Seattle, but she couldn't tell me why; it was a secret. She then told me about all the murals she was making. Her ideas continued to move, quickly, without much of a connection. I worried about her and called Dad. He flew to Olympia three days later. When Dad came she screamed at him and kept the doors locked."*

This psychotic episode was many times worse than the episode at Macalester. Her illness had progressed, and a schizophrenia like psychosis was now mixed in with manic-depression. This was a horrific experience for Dorie who wrote a partial description of her experience:

> *'The scenery changes abruptly and I am staring out the splintered window of my home in Olympia, Washington and into the star-smattered sky. Jutting out from the window are an empty aluminum foil tube, a broom and a few patches of saran wrap to cover up the jagged edges of the broken window. It is a night SETI would be proud of. Peering through my cardboard telescope I have seen through the fabric of space-time itself,*

ridden the wrinkles of time on my broom while standing still splashing raspberry yogurt onto my floor with ecstatic strokes. Jonah is an entrapment delusion. I am a traveler unstuck in time."

It was also horrific for the rest of us to see evidence of what Dorie had experienced. Mary wrote about what she saw:

"There were shrines all over her trailer and out on the lawn; candles, pictures cut from National Geographic's, records, clothing. She had thrown books on the lawn that sat for days, ruined by the rain. She set fire to a Mola, a stitched piece of work, originally crafted to be a blouse, by women who lived on the San Blas Islands off Panama. Dad liked to collect them and Dorie always admired them growing up. He gave one to her as a special gift. She let it burn inside the stove. She shaved off all her hair."

7

I have the utmost respect for the mental health community in Olympia. After my call they acted quickly to move Dorie from her home to, for the third time in her life, a locked ward in a hospital. The psychiatrist at the hospital was direct with Dorie. He told her that she needed to take the most medication she could tolerate. Otherwise he said each new episode would be worse than the preceding one.

Before this, mental health professionals seemed unwilling to emphasize the seriousness of her illness to Dorie and her family. Perhaps it only became clear over time as the full pattern emerged. Now the diagnosis was clearly schizoaffective disorder, a mixture of schizophrenia and bipolar disorder. Each of these chronic mental illnesses is very serious, and the combination even more so.

After Dorie was discharged from the hospital in the spring of 2000, I flew again to Olympia. We packed some of her things into her car and hired a moving company to move the rest and together drove home to Duluth. Sometime later she accused me of kidnaping her. While this was not entirely correct I felt strongly that Dorie living alone so far away from her family was simply not realistic or safe.

Back in Duluth, Dorie continued her college work through Evergreen. She graduated and received a Bachelor of Arts degree. Given all she faced this was a significant achievement! Yet she was not proud of it because she believed her final work at Evergreen was not up to her standard of excellence.

By the summer of 2000 Dorie was feeling better and decided to travel to Peru on an educational program. But something about that trip went badly for her, and she flew home after only one day in Peru. By this point in her life even when feeling well the illness had eroded her ability to cope with adversity.

8

A RESPITE in DULUTH
With Subsequent Psychotic Episode

The time period between 2000 and 2001 was mostly productive for Dorie. She wrote more poems during this time than any other time. From that time period Mary and I both have memories of Dorie having fun, smiling and laughing, at least for short times. Mary wrote:

> "I keep the image of Dorie and me playing soccer together down at the cabin with our younger cousins. She was running and laughing as we all chased after the ball, kicking each other's shins and creating the boundaries as we went."

Her fourth psychotic episode was starting late summer 2001. One day I went to visit her. She was lying in bed. After a short conversation Dorie told me she had swallowed an entire bottle of pills. She said she needed relief from the terrible things going on in her head. I called 911. A doctor told me that the pills would not have killed her, but would have made her very sick. That event seemed to be a wakeup call for the mental health people in Duluth.

After a short hospital stay in Duluth Dorie was transferred to a mental health long term care facility in Eveleth, Minnesota. The purpose for Dorie to be in this facility was to find a mix of medications that could keep her healthy. The process of finding the best medications for her was basically one of trial and error. The psychiatrist tried the least bothersome medications first and kept going with more difficult medications as he found that nothing worked for her. Finally he tried the strongest and most troublesome medication available. That worked, but left Dorie with side effects. The process took several months and Dorie was at Eveleth until January 2002.

While in the hospital Dorie wrote Mary a letter:

> *"In communication we are raised to believe that most transactions take place between individuals face to face, or by some other media like phone, fax, music, artwork, etc. I have been taking on psychic relays enough to drive anyone crazy, and more than enough for someone who already is. I don't need to know what celebrity X is doing if I think of that person more than I need a tail. Anyway my transgressions and my wrong thinking have magnified so large there is very little of me left. My mind is a slushy compost pile, like we talked about, waiting to push up begonias.*

9

"I find myself grappling for defense on all the wrong avenues, like involuntary insults or inappropriate thoughts that I really don't mean. Just when I think things are under control these things are taken from my mind, leaving me in a state of constant panic as to what will surface next. I am perpetually more than "one down" everywhere I go; I don't know how to climb back up. It is maddening. This is not me, not what I have ever been. For reasons outside of my control, my mind has become my worst enemy."

A few weeks before she was discharged from Eveleth Dorie wrote:

There is a cozy catholic church down the street that I visit irregularly. Praying the rosary gives me some peace of mind (as opposed to a mind of pieces)."

Her Final Chapter

After Dorie returned home from Eveleth in January 2002 she lived on her own and tried to keep herself busy. She continued to write poetry, visit Hannah House and volunteered at the food shelf. She worked at various part time jobs. Dorie and I spent a lot of time together. We walked the Lakewalk in Duluth several times a week in good weather and bad. We had a Sunday routine of church and then lunch. At other times we went to Subway for a sandwich. We often just went out for a meal together. Given what followed, I'm grateful for this time we had together.

As another episode was starting Dorie wrote six poems in the last two days of her life. They provide some insight into the state of her mind then. Three of those poems are included in this book:

"I walk a thin line" (Page 28) "snares" (Page 29) "Channels benign begin" (Page 30)

July 18, 2003 was a beautiful summer day. Dorie, driving alone, died instantly in an automobile accident. The relief she wanted from the terrible, horrible, and debilitating things going on in her head occurred at that instant. Our family's grief over her loss started.

Actually, that was just the final loss. We had lost her, bit by bit, over many years—exactly as she had lost herself.

A bench on the Duluth Lakewalk was dedicated to Dorie. Her poem "she is a yellow butterfly" (Page 65) is included on the dedication plaque attached to the bench.

11

Mental Health Lessons Learned

This story and Dorie's poetry emphasize that patients and their loved ones need better early understanding of mental illness to mitigate cascading seriousness of the illness. A few lessons that may be learned from Dorie's experience are:

• Don't expect mental health systems to be as helpful as you need them to be.

• Mental health systems focus on patients and not on families of patients.

• An early and accurate diagnosis is essential, but may not be clear until the full pattern of the illness evolves over time.

• Yet waiting for the full pattern to emerge wastes the opportunity for early and persistent treatment to prevent avoidable worsening.

• Patients need early, ongoing, and persistent care.

• Families need early, ongoing and persistent education and support.

• Patients and families need early, ongoing and persistent advocacy.

• The importance of finding and always taking medications that work cannot be over emphasized to prevent further destructive episodes.

• The importance of consistently taking medication even when feeling better cannot be over emphasized. Rather than "I feel better, so I can stop taking the medication," be thankful it is working and *keep taking it.* Medications for mental illness may take some time to start working effectively. Everyone needs to be patient and give them time to work.

• The capacity needed to best cope with the illness is markedly impaired during episodes, and even more as the illness progresses with each new episode.

• Each new psychotic episode takes something away from the patient's personality that never returns.

• Yet, at least for Dorie, in periods between episodes her insight and ability to write about her illness was not impaired.

• If only Dorie had received an early, accurate diagnosis; if only we had been told sooner that each new psychotic episode would be worse than the previous one; if only Dorie and we, her family, had been told sooner that she needed to take the maximum amount of medication she could tolerate; if only we had been told that each new episode would take something away from the person Dorie had been that never would return; if only Dorie and we had been told all of these things... then the course of her illness may have been considerably less severe.

Professional Review
Of Dorie's Poetry

We are greatly indebted to Myriam J. A. Chancy, Ph.D. for reviewing and providing a description of Dorie's poetry. Dr. Chancy earned her Ph.D. in English. She is an award winning writer, college professor having held tenure-track positions at several universities and is Hartley Burr Alexander Chair in the Humanities at Scripps College of the Claremont Colleges. She has a long list of publications including seven books and several academic monographs. She is a frequently invited guest speaker nationally and internationally and serves as an expert reviewer for professional journals, university presses and tenure-promotion reviews nationally.

In excerpts from her review Dr. Chancy said:

"Reading the work chronologically, one notes that the choice is increasingly assured and one can observe a movement from prose poems to minimalist poetry signaling the formation of a distinct style. The poet makes liberal use of nature imagery to convey psychological and emotional states in ways that are compelling for the reader." *The most solid work is that which deals with the author's illness that appears to have occupied*

much of her emotional and creative concerns, for obvious reasons; then, the more experimental work (the "magnetic" poems and other haiku-like poems) also stand out as having aesthetic integrity of their own."

Myriam Chancy categorized the poems based on related themes into eight groupings. The groupings in her words are: "1) magnetic poems; 2) Spanish poems; 3) narrative or prose poems; 4) love poems; 5) early poems (in different styles—though of interest, most read like class exercises); 6) minimalist "nature" poetry; 7) "erotic" poetry; 8) first person poems (most longer) on illness."

She then rearranged the poems and selected 62 of the most compelling poems and three short prose pieces from 125 pages of Dorie's collected work. She placed the poems in four sections to suggest a comprehensive order. That is the order poems are presented in this book. They are not in chronological order except for Section 3 about Magnetic Poetry which she said, "for some reason, these work in chronological order as a group from oldest to most recent."

Enjoy this work from a beautiful, intelligent, creative, talented, caring, and committed person—she was worth knowing and the poems are worth reading.

With all my love for my daughter, Dorie,

Bob Reichert
Duluth, MN
Autumn 2020

14

16

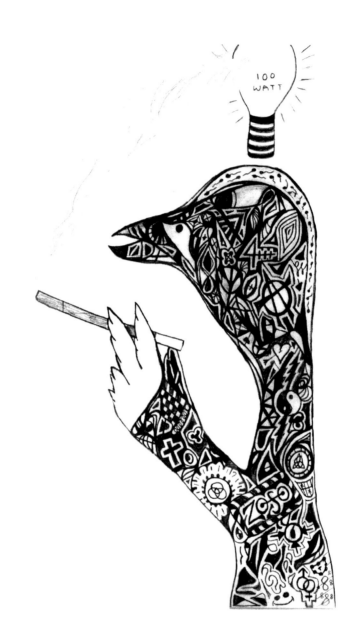

Section One:
Manic Depression

17

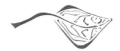

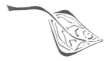

18

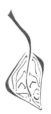

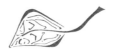

Manic Depression

M
 a
  n
   i
    c
     D
      e
       p
        r
       e
        s
         s
         i
         o
         n

The letters
      drop from my mouth
          like dominoes
             falling
clink!
     crash!
       bang!

a pile on my floor

I try to pick the letters up,
to reform those words
and reestablish order
out of all this entropy

         but of course
               it is a trick
               order out of entropy
               still spelling out
               disorder

                  11/5/96
                  DJR

19

When I Fall

Alice's wonderland occupies a permanent space in my mind. You could say I fall mto a black hole when I travel, that all other realities fade away. You could also say that I escape from a black hole when I travel, that my mind becomes like a universal sigularity bursting from some unknown to rearrange the known universe of mind... When I open my eyes though, I sit staring not in my favorite chair with a cat named Dinah in my lap, but at the cosmically and terrestrially challenged battlefield of my life. I see it through a new kaleidoscope of mind each time, in a vision that has made the past, the present, and the future into a colorfully fragmented wheel spinning constantly before me.

20

When I fall. I fall not into a rabbit hole, but through a portal in my own mind that combines every moment I have ever lived with every moment I have ever imagined. To live the dream and call it reality and never really be free from the vehicle that took me there? What is that? And how do I know when I'm awake?

silver sea

silver sea
magnanimity
this gravity
taken from me

tune-space
illusions of confusion
disillusion
I would efface all these
dissolution

time-space
I split the light
kaleidoscopic mind
eternity
quaternity
a picture parsed
from one singularity
spirits one all
bound transcendent
in the bittersweet
enigma of reality

DJR
8/31/01

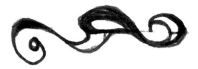

It is a March Midwestern Night

It is a March midwestern night and frost threatens to edge its way across my windshield. Inside my body, I feel the bass coming from the warehouse behind me as though it were sounding out of my chest. The music pulses not only out of that building, but out of me. Somewhere there is an invisible conduit that channels the messages in beats per minute between me and the source. The beat is a language, a mathematical code of intensity designed to emit messages to a higher intelligence. No one in the car seems to understand this but me.

For the last twenty minutes. I have been watching a monorail-like train pass back and forth on the tracks in front of the parking lot. With images from the movie *Contact* fresh in my mind, it occurs to me that this might be my ship, my gateway to another dimension. Abruptly I slip from the driver's seat and out into the fading night. The white cars shimmer in the distance. I picture myself inside one of them, flying along at the speed of light until the tracks disappear and I am Jodi Foster moving through the wormholes of space. Destination: the unknown Universe. Non-stop. No-return. Back to stardust, as Carl Sagan might say. I am ready.

***

It is a long road home.

sun at high noon

sun at high noon
spreading the mist
leaving a space
for my shadow to walk

DJR
10/24/01

23

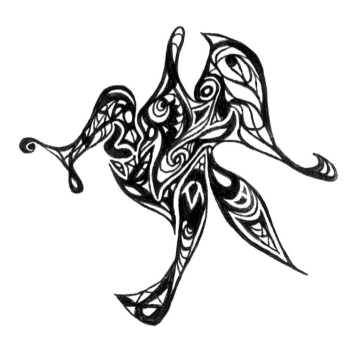

i walk a thin line

i walk a thin line
between two worlds
one of flesh and spirit
the other of decay and ghosts
narrow in path
i cannot flee
or desist
from its specter
i walk a thin line

24

DJR
7/16/03

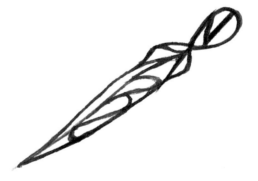

snares

snares
are set
all around
this mountain
flourishing green
nets to trap
wires to snare
agile i would be
but for minds own decay
snares
are set
all around
this mountain
flourishing green

7/17/03
DJR

25

channels benign begin

channels bening begin
trickles of words
then arrives
the violent maelstrom
oceans of thoughts
pouring onto my shore
tide
waxing and waning
in conspicuous give and take
consciousness a wreath
i would not wear for long

DJR
7/17/03

26

temper frustration angst

temper frustration angst
a pang from the past
juvenile undertow
dark currents
alight in my waking hour
memory
the illusion of tranquility
in season's first snow
smoke curling skyward
my hand reaching out to greet
the familiar unfamiliar
like two trains passing
on parallel tracks
frozen rails
for a course

DJR
10-24-01

27

phosphor incandescence

phosphor incandescence
lights a starless path
new moon
concealer of shadows
memory
a knotted branch
failing
in the direction
of high snows

11/16/01
DJR

28

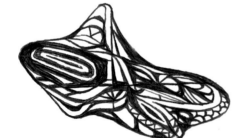

new moon

new moon
frantic storm
sleep remains
like a heavy goodbye

dream a dream
perfect silence
cool against
their broken words
one will retreat
into nothing
shame for a token

12/5/01
DJR

29

accusations

accusations
bearing
false witness
a nickel for
a wrong word
turned right
sour fruit
serves a withered
tree
memory a blunt edge
against night's comet
burning bright
across the sky

11/16/01
DJR

30

midnight star

midnight star
abdicate
your constellation
for you
time cuts a path
interstellar
fall away
desist
and
be gone
like one sure comet
burning fast
into future's
extremity

11/27/01
DJR

31

twilight star

twilight star
evemng rise
soft over the shoulder
of afternoon's
cold sun
nested fast
in winter's
bonnet

1/4/02
DJR

32

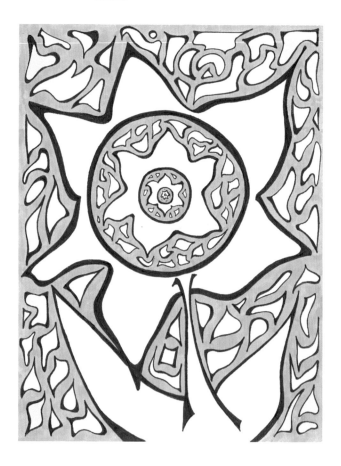

fifty blossoms

fifty blossoms
a sovereign constellation
a flag draped on an olive branch
Gethsemenie
a state of sorrow
a place of grace
a garden
transmutation
a higher state of consciousness
Zion's doors open in every nation

33

10/24/01
DJR

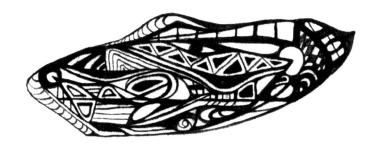

temperance

temperance
a contemplative lull
buried in the skin
of yesteryear
dizzying spells
of the morrow
laid aside
to gather
their own furtive faints
for raw surfacing

DJR
1/23/02

34

<u>mind</u>

    mind
    a fertile wasteland
    mutinous metronome
    keeps the time
    grievous upheaval
    saboteur plays the fool

    10/28/01
    DJR

35

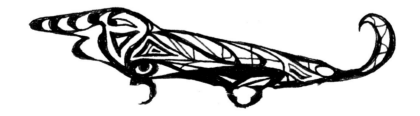

passion flame

passion flame
spark
in the night
cool shadow
walks amidst
the glow
heat
untempered

DJR
4/20/03

36

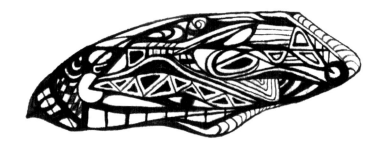

solar undertaker

solar undertaker
breathes
wings of fire
transporting
cold stalagmite
miner's hands
raw surfacing
noontide thaw
squinting at the light
cavemen unite
this flame is a purge
of old
ashes ashes
come dance 'round
a promise
of tomorrow
heat on our backs

11/8/01
DJR

flashdance

the rod comes down
happenstance
cursed inheritance
I see in my own temperament
a small edge
sharpened
of my Father's lance

DJR
11/5/01

38

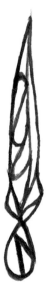

interdisciplinary disciple

interdisciplinary disciple
jagged fragment
of a violent syncretism
mind a gray painting
poured open
out onto the canvas
of the world
there
in that fine art
my love is
a corpulent strain
left best for beggars
and thieves
my church a sad fixture
of hypocrisy or
an indifferent opiate
in a long game of chase
that would hardly seem
to retire my shadow
courage palled over
by imperfection broadcast
strength a mobius rebound
on high

11/10/01
DJR

39

machinations

machinations
grind
a modern axis
turning
on
conflagration
a grating of
steel on steel
hard drums
tolling fast
a quickened
appetite
for
destruction

11/12/01
DJR

40

fury

fury
a familiar rod
drives an acute flame
scorched earth
destitute plane

11/28/01
DJR

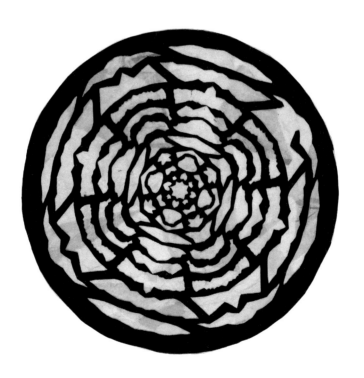

frantic sky

frantic sky
hometown remains
loud moments
tight visions
dream a dirty whine
storm remaining

12/9/01

42

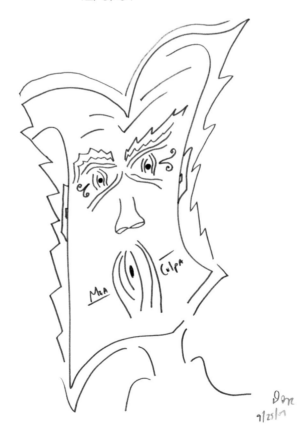

harbor mist

harbir mist
envelope me
with your chill
cold arms
seething embrace
harbor mist

DJR
7/17/03

43

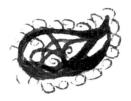

44

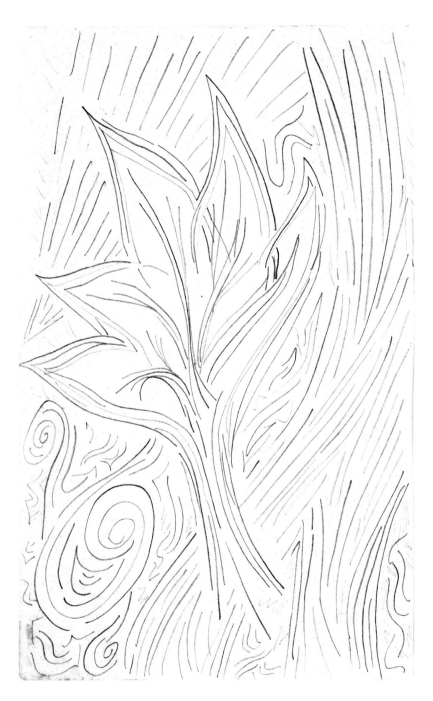

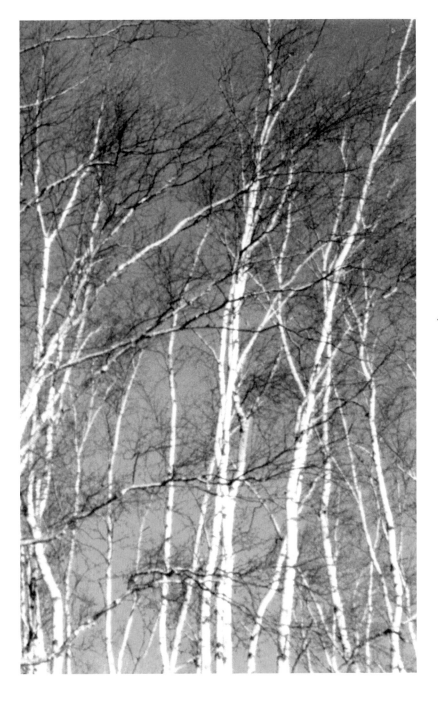

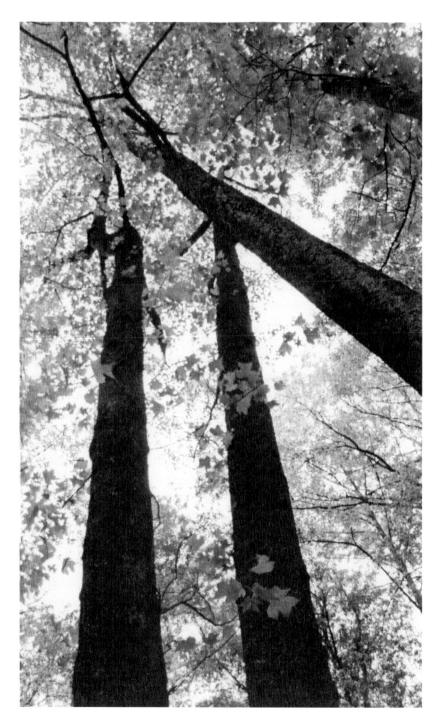

46

Section Two:
Oceans of Words

47

oceans of words

oceans of words
weavte their way
through my waking hours
threading seeds of contempt
bitter pills
mirrors ajar
for crooked reflection
how i would have my mind
be a sharpened lance
and not a soft bruised fruit
decaying slowly
awash in oceans of words
oceans of words

DJR
7/16/03

Insanity

a seed that lurks
in the mind
flowering in the season
of its own despair

DJR
5/20/98

49

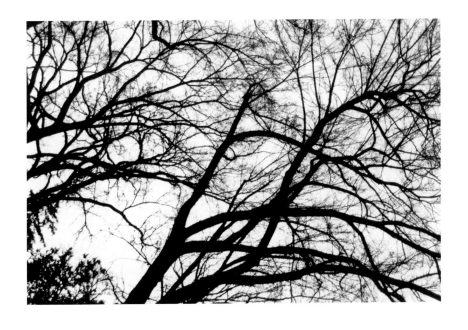

Purpose

purpose
this thing that I purport—
she supposes herself
in a pose,
the poise
of a porpoise
or perhaps
a syrupy posy
of purple roses

I am sore
rumpled and pulpy
and she eros
dumplings and lupines

50

Supine
I lay like a marsupial
smarmy and pursed
at the lips
slipping like a lisp
from my own mouth
spilling
willing
fulfilling
this syrupy
purple
promise
with
lupine
poise

DJR 5/1/99

the day passes like fog

the day passes like fog over a city... i am looking through the crystal of my mind and seeing the prism of my surroundings refracted at an angle through my thoughts

mind
a pyramid
diffused
with light
prism
a spectrum
piercing
the mind
color
a
day
leaving
this temple
fog
the shadow
of
interpretation

5/13/99
DJR

51

12:00 AM

12:00 AM midnight coils smooth calm sky roiling summer frost against my skin

king cobra
spiral might
coiled tight
desire a hiss
despair a shudder

beats lick my neck
a steady pulse
coursing submerged
in time

falling
like an accent
over nascent
footsteps
intent a scale
repentance a maelstrom

winding thru galactic arms
held in
held out
taken from within
taken from without

formless
i am formed

spiral scales
and midnight air
a universe within
a universe
an accent falling
over troubled time

DJR 7/17/99

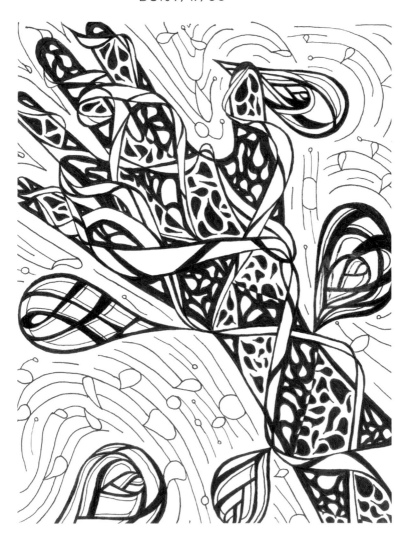

death beckons

deaht beckons
this shrill whispering sister
armed like a shadow
falling from the temple of spirit—
she walks with me
yet
I do not know her;
her face a mirror
to my own
she has held me
since the crisis of living
poured open my mind
and splintered my soul,
since the dark river
birthed my body
into the 1ight
and since
the tide of time
first began—

it was in broken consciousness
that the tremors first seized—

grown
I grasped like a child
for her elusive shape,
a cold seething sorrow
wed unto me
this uninvited hand
bearing veiled promises,
stirring and soothing,
watching silent
as the tiles rung chill
beneath my feet

why do you come to me like this?
rushing
the gates of an acute nerve
to flood the senses
with your bittersweet taste?
I do not measure the hours
cannot count the minutes

is it for you
that I ought make the minutes
count?

55

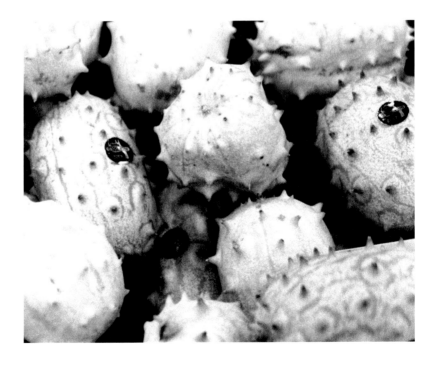

<u>cloaked in terror</u>

cloaked in terror
your sentence
is but a declaration

turned exclamation

the crisis

a revelation
of violent
and abundant
beauty

DJR
11/25/99

56

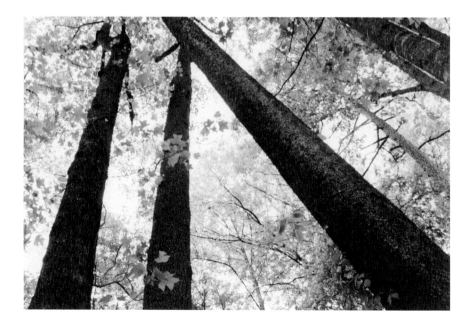

black dreams

black dreams
would incubate
silent screams
still
like the sorrow
of hurricane dreams

eye
the storm
calm amidst chaos
chaos amidst calm

a frenetic well
pools
I
this well
without walls
barricading
walls without a well

the source
shivers
grows cold
a child speaks
with aged eyes
I a storm
pooling sorrow
unfurling
like
a stream steady

running
chasing eyes
running fast
to avert
the source
of sorrow

black dreams
silent screams
running

I chase ahead
look behind
close my eyes
pretending
I can fly

58

no more will
I die
each day
a passing moment
of another
dull play

my dreams
the subject
of abject
scrutiny

silently
I scream
holding myself tight
with needful foresight

I did not ask
for the stars
to shine like this
at night

tomorrow I see
another plight

clock fixed
eternally
on midnight

DJR
3/10/00

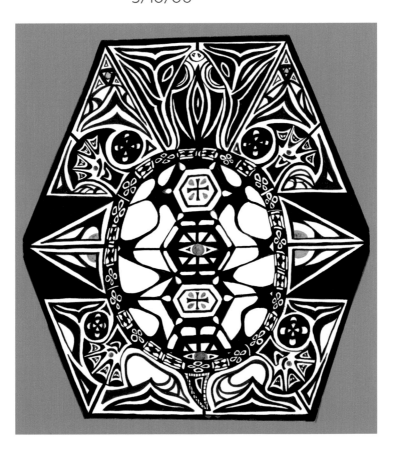

siren's bells

siren's bells
florid like a manic day
crashing Doplar
FX tuning on high

a rock i would have
my body be
strength in its formidable
tomb
that none would travel

i cry out
as metal on metal
splits a double
at the hands of God

my fist
an impotent tool
i cannot raise

DJR
10/3/01

60

a tired eye winds

a tired eye winds
nave spells rushing
evil
do dispell

this sorcerer's hand
Crowley haunts
the gates
of my mind
turning sweet to bitter
deficit of hope to faith

illusion a swarming
tsunami rising
in a tide of true believers
chanting hollow tunes

a withered flower
for an offering

10/3/01
DJR

a twisted skein is woven

a twisted skein is woven
mistakes threaded
in deference to God
a fabric of necessity
to know better
of his perfect way

I wear my exquisite shall
with pride
and wrap it with his grace

the better I become
for these flaws
as I witness the quickening
of his love
drawing closer

DJR
9.13.01

she is a yellow butterfly

she is a yellow butterfly
cocooned in time
sad like a dark song
crying to fly

DJR
3/98

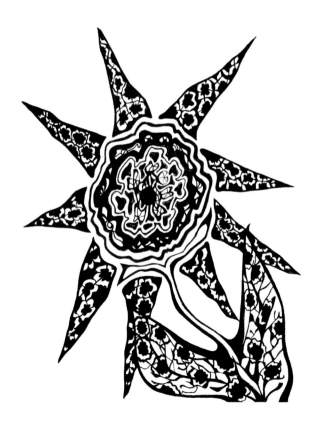

red tide rising

red tide rising
black star falls back
behind the curtain
a sparrow sings a high note
sunbeam for a nest
the oceans drum the shores
of time
black star fall back
behind this uni-spectral filter
consciousness
a new moonbeam
a hearkened cry
drought of paradise
cleaving to my soul

DJR
10-24-01

64

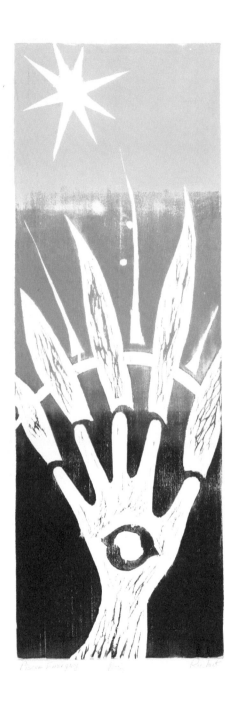

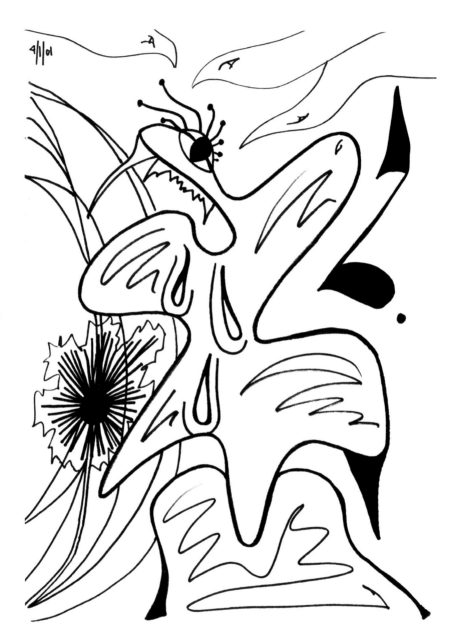

66

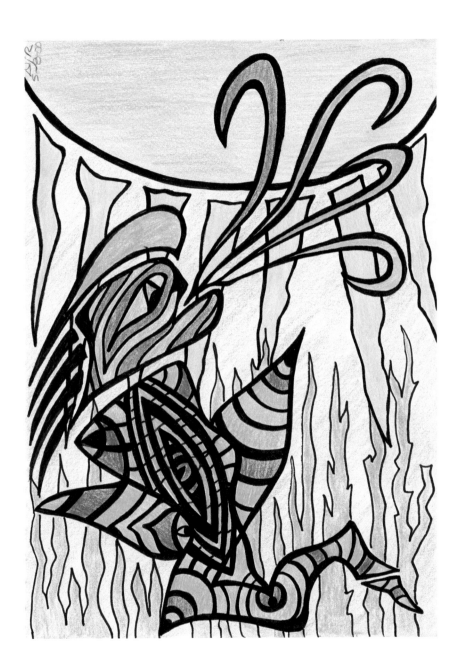

67

68

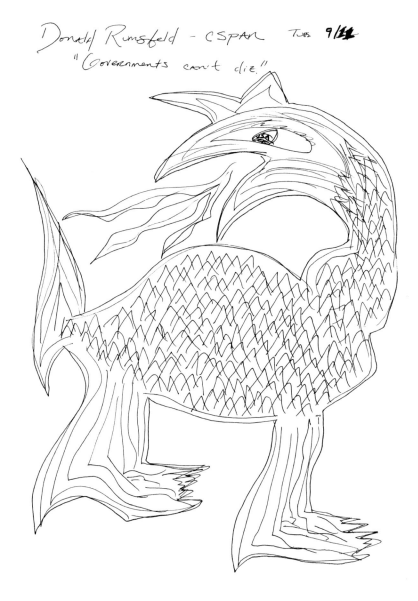

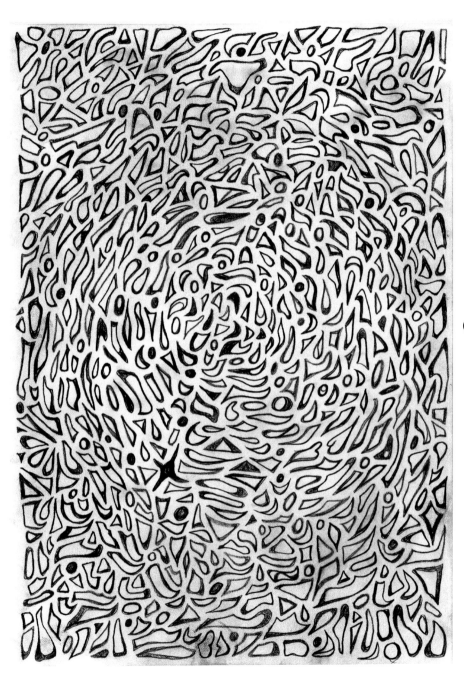

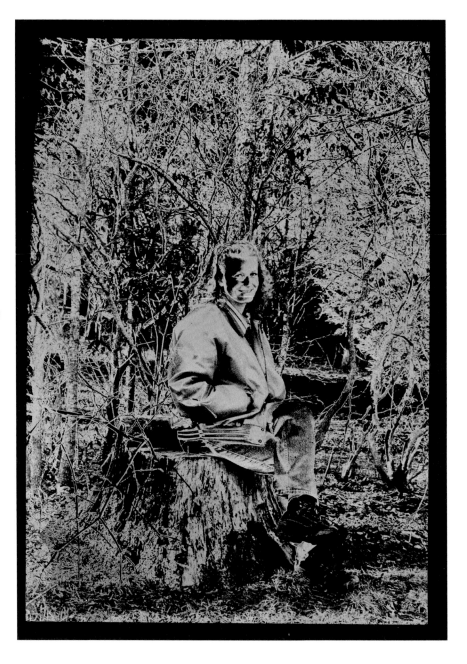

Section Three:
Magnetic Poetry

71

72

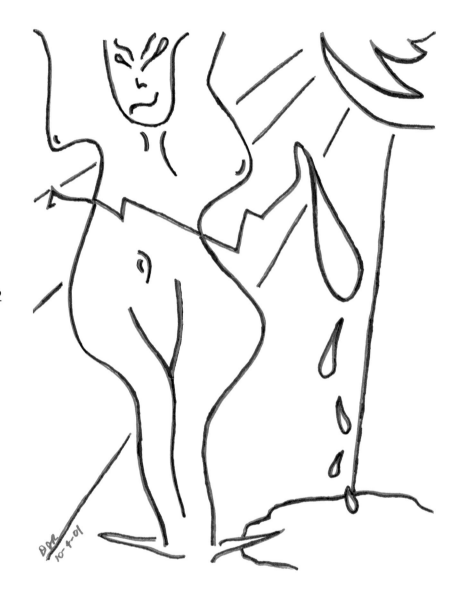

magnetic, woman

woman

smooth arms
butt
breasts

she is honey

ugly hair
repulsive goddess

drunk
delicate
gorgeous peach

delirious with need

11/10/96
DJR

73

magnetic, winter storm

winter storm
blowing
diamonds
from
the
sky

74

sad man
still like a thousand white moments
summer a shadow

11/10/96
DJR

magnetic, eggy

magnetic.eggy rosehip moon on a heavy summer night
egg
moon
heaveing languidly
whispering
summer

do you recall the rain (?]

luscious & blue

like
hot rose petal juice
smeared over my tongue

11/10/96
DJR

magnetic, eternity

a languid shadow shines still
under a cool winter moon

eternity

a raining symphony of light
there beneath the crushing blue sky

12/97
DJR

magnetic, trip

stop these
rusty red
diamond trips
and lather me
in iron

7/99
DJR

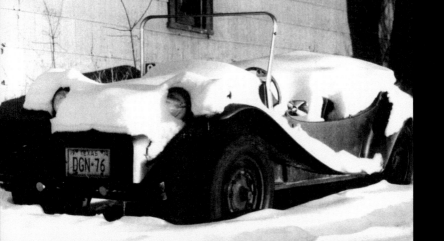

the magnetic soothsayer

bitter day
ask forested voids
chanting like winter
what may play
next

here a beat
ugly storm
cool like sea mist

place a smell
78
sweet with yellow sleep

who yet goes to tell

drunk in recalling
the blue smear
honey moon
black sun

shining
like summer light
falling
over iron feet

8/99
DJR

magnetic, lick some honey

lick some honey
she hits moon mist

sun & chocolate
would incubate black dreams
white like the screaming mother

love crushing

79

his gift

time the road light a knife

a fiddle at her feet

DJR
8/19/99

80

magnetic, summer

swim falling
sad like a knife

pink rose
frantic woman

run over me
shaking

road an elaborate
red chain

cool beneath
drunken whispers

and white produce

smell an elaborate suit

music a black rainy language

crushing bitter breasts

DJR
3/8/00

magnetic, storm

repulsive petal
watch the rain

lazy symphony
always a sleepy moon

what lather soars
whispered blue blood

heaving
I licked through men

a friendly cry
boiling like said ships

sun a sausage TV
luscious void
delirious winter
shining
moments

picture these
recall the raw day

sky a gift

DJR
3/8/00

smooth shadow
road the essential mother
languid eternity
she cool like death
goes waxing time
and want
flooding my summer
with still wind
and weak aching
moments

5/27/00
DJR

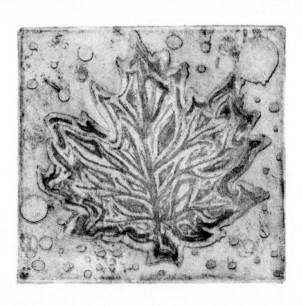

magnetic.life

after

behind

next

was

is

5/27/00

DJR

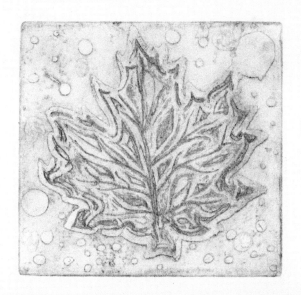

84

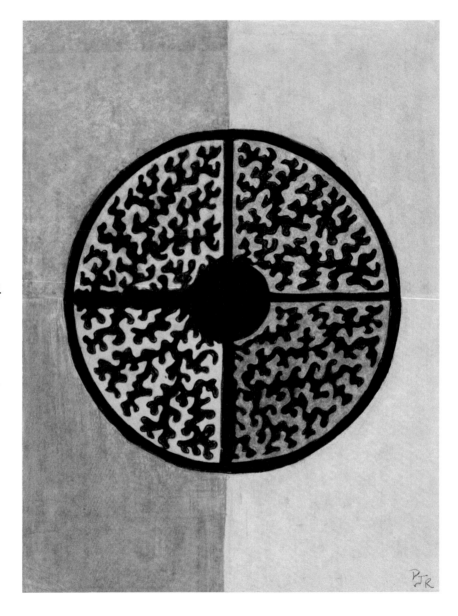

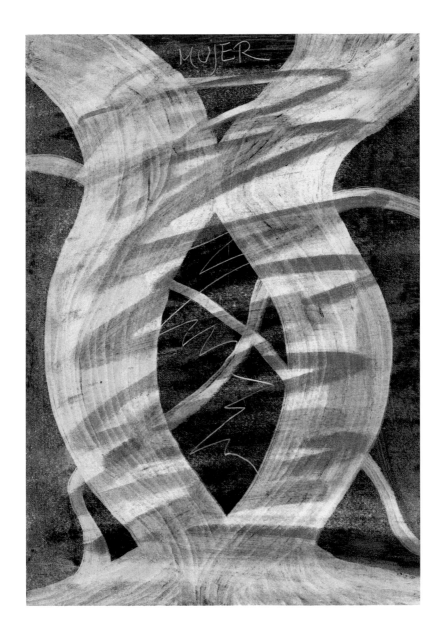

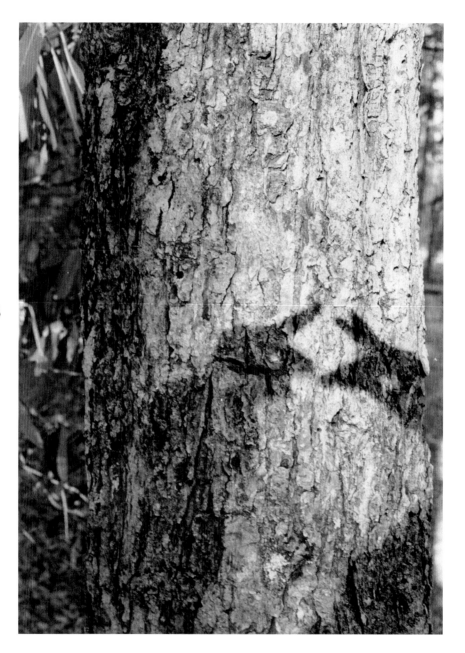

Section Four:
i want to live the anarchy

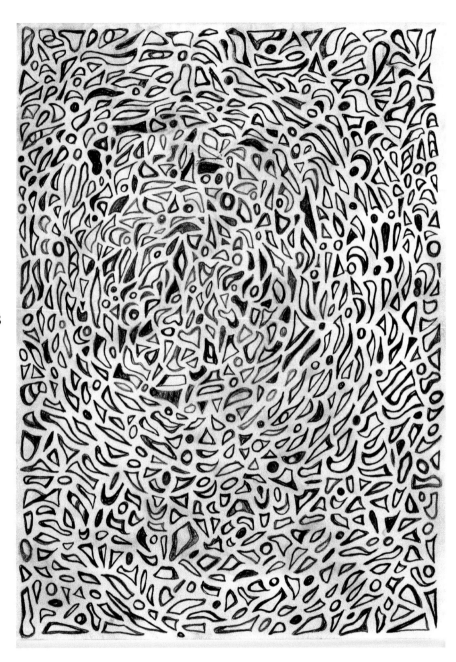

i want to live the anarchy

i want to live the anarchy of self in a governed sphere
        can love be my law?
        be still in fury
        be fury in stillness

        live the higher mind
        guard the earthly gates
        from the blunt swords of deceit
        hone the blade of integrity

        and reap

        8/18/99

89

Mother Always Told Me

Mother Always Told Me Not To Rub My Eyes
When I close my eyes
Clenched fists against lids
Surrender to the pitch of black,
And so I soar behind a curtain
of darkness,
Watching tesselations triumph over absence—
Turning, shifting, morphing—
Rapt, my mind's eye
A giant screen saver
Hosting
Flying toasters
that drift shiftless and content
Through a hapless programmed chaos—

Here,
I dream of you
My unbuttered love
And sing such odiferous odes
Of nonsensical nothings
As to inspire the capricious flapping
Of those perfect white wings
Against the burned screen of my eyes.

3/20/95
DJR

the repulsive dress

the repulsive dress
ugly and languid
mad blood beneath
run away frantic
aching like some essential lie
ugly and true
she's part urges and beauty
no easy woman

DJR
2/3/0 l

91

Pegasus, Celestial Body

She wears Orion's belt
snug around her waist
And keeps the Big Dipper
by the bath
for when it's off

The Seven Sisters all say
She's not so heavenly
that she burned out long ago
   but Orion swears
   she is his Pegasus
and rides her through the night
just to show them so.

11/18/96
DJR

desert moon

desert moon
rising languid

slow over Tuscon hills

11/18/96
DJR

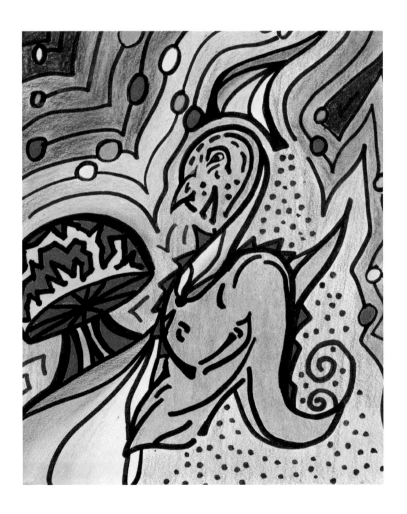

<u>69</u>

lips
butts
breasts
a mi me tocan tus manos
y a ti te hago lo mismo

arriba
abajo
asi se mueven (las manos)
groping
pulling
up/and/then/down/the
steady undulating slope
of our bodies
hands tracing each curve
mi seis
conforming to your nine
tu nueve
cradling the curve
of my six

Aqui estamos
un gigante nudo desnudo
cradled and sucking like babies
en eso que nos ha hecho

11/26/96
DJR

94

Erotic Margarita

Erotic Margarita
You came to me
                    Frozen
But luckily
        I knew what to do

One hand
        curled
around your chic
                glassy curves

My mouth
        wrapped
over your smooth
                unexpecting
                        lip
Slowly
    I rocked you
towards me
            until suddenly

I had you in my mouth
sweet and runny
sour green slush

explosive ecstacy

pouring
    down
        my
            throat

11/18/96
DJR

95

DIANA

Pale
luna
she is silver
a soft celestial eye
casting moonray tides
through the starry night

12/12/96
DJR

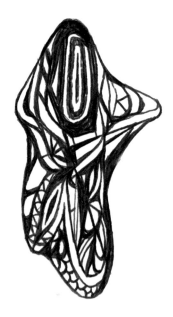

harvest moon rising

harvest moon rising
earth's curve a smooth trembling lip
on the lunar horizon

10/97
DJR

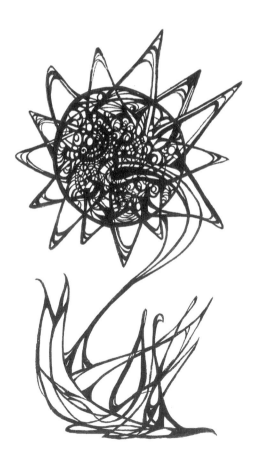

summer

three months and another crease
in your sheets
is how I count the days of summer—
white linen draped over your curves,
I fold myself into the creases
of your body
like the sheets that cover us,
pulling you over me
for warmth

10/21/97
DJR

98

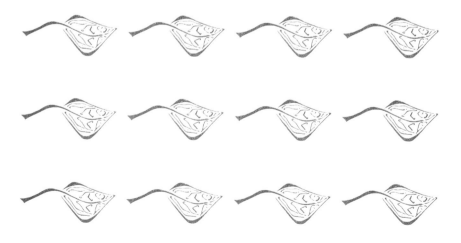

No one ever thinks about

no one ever thinks about
the orange—
plump thick-skinned pilgrim
who comes to us in winter.
bewildered,
summer dripping fresh from its flesh
like warm citrus tears
soon to be licked and forgotten.

11-18-97
DJR

99

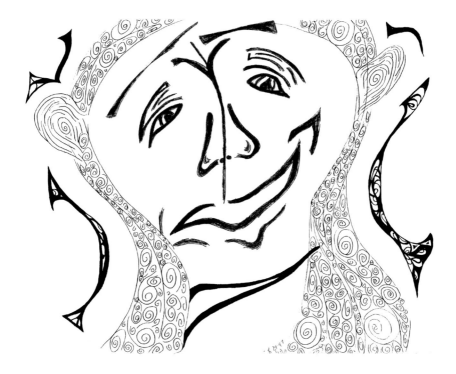

she sketches lines

she sketches lines
smooth straight winding
transfonnations
inking rivers
that spill over flat sheet valleys
uncovering
a mythic geography
a dragon suspended
in a sun-streaked sky
flowers unfolding underhand
here
space speaks balance
white jockeying black
lines conjoined
to round an edge
or thicken a wall

soon a figure will emerge

6/13/97 (Revised 8/20/99)
DJR

I once dreamed that my body

I once dreamed that my body
was made of sponge and that
I could absorb the oceans
around me

plankton and jellyfish
slipping past sediment
and sharks' teeth

coral reefs left standing like
old desert bones

101

salt and saline
tears and ocean swelling as one
settling with the midnight moon

all that I am made of
swimming inside
one heavy sponge
bowed by its own weight
for want to be wrung

DJR
7/19/98

swimmer

her love cuts like a blunt knife,
slow and rough—
but men need her bed,
lusting for her sad hair
or a place to put away
their faded pictures
of a woman long ago loved

she is a picture now too,
an old familiar face that cries
in a locket she cannot open—
pierced once by love,
she hides her heart
away in the shallow folds
of men who do not love her

taking their pain she bears down,
cutting hers free—
she thinks the wounds will close
this way,
sutured by sweat and tight embraces
that slip away fast
like water through her hands

1/24/98
DJR

Norshor June 21

hips like goldfish
honey hair streaming like a sea
of charmed snakes
she swims across the floor
slithering to the beat and
keeping time in her waist
forehead shimmering
under a spotlight sunset
sweat running salty
down her cheeks

6/21/97
DJR

103

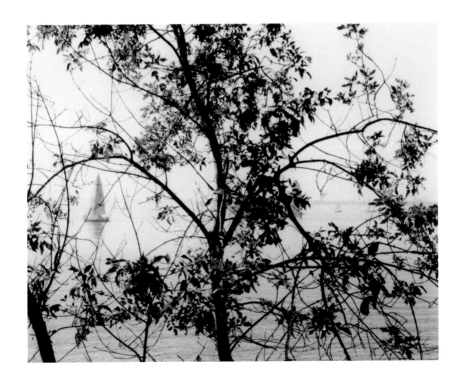

three days

three days
and my lips are parted
like two soft and supple shores
missing the ocean
of your kiss

12/97
DJR

104

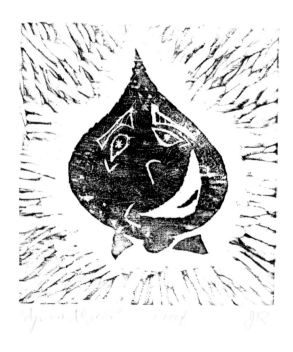

morning

silver dawn streaks the horizon

cool Earth
a tranquil blossoming flame—

hands spread like the new light,
I swallow the color.
temper this heat—
a flower opens

and a new day dawns

3/27/97
O.JR

105

ai tin

ai tin
la justicia y yo
encuentrense
en una batalla
de lluvia

un dia frio
morfre aquello dia
un flor sucio
volando en las alas
de la eternidad
ser con dios
el creador de mundos
inconceble
el padre de toda gente
v el juez doloroso del mi alma

l 0/6/01
DJR

Shoot the moon.

Anything standing still, spinning fast, ordinary and elusive with a shadow to bear. My heart becomes an arrow and with the drawstring I pull back slow and calculating, reaping all the sorrow and violence that gravity would pull from her orbit into my own. Insight, the subconscious pulse of existence ringing like a symphonic maelstrom in my mind, and the mottled beauty of my soul are gifts I release with a quick sling. This cold fire that would burn me I transform and Hermes, the messenger arrow of my heart, quickens through space. With a jolt the blazing tip pierces the silvery cratered luminescence of the moon. The flame I carry, this tenuous dance between Eros and Thanos, recoils into its native soil. But I know she will kindle it with the tides and everything in her orbit will come back to me in time. I draw another arrow and she smiles like the Venus de Milo, but when she turns about I see her shadow. I cry out and pull the sands beneath me through my hands. Soon the tides will draw high again and my hean will pulse with new undercurrents. She will send me new moonshadows kindled from the ashes of old. Thanos at one tum and Eros at another, laughing together at the magnificence of their own dance and the prospect of a conscious partner. Thanos would like to have me for himself, a shadow player stirring the well and lifting the tides ever higher. Eros loves him and when I dance with her I am pulled even then by his influence. She twirls me through things that are green and soft and supple like tamarak or the nape of yesterday's neck. She is Goya's maja desnuda in Nathaniel Hawthorne's secret garden, tantalizing and radiant with the smell of sweetgrass and honeydew, yet incomplete without the shadow of death at her side.

107

Perhaps I could be writing the story of my soul pierced to ashes and rising again like the phoenix. Come close and, like the moon, I will pull at the tides of your subconscious, shifting sediments and filling you with a mixture of curiosity and ambivalence or even desire and disgust. Maybe your own tide of being thinks I could unveil for you some mystery that has pierced me but that is latent in you. Some promise of renewal seen radiant in the glow of illusion, one that shrouds violence in beauty, death in art. Maybe you do not want to know the soul's arduous story of renewal, transcendence and grace. You revile commotion, disorder, confusion, and pain, and when you glimpse a story you know well in me you feel afraid. I am not gentle like the moon because my mind has been split open too many times. So really I am only busy shooting arrows into the night sky and crying for the lovers in the garden and for the bitter sweetness of a world that can't live without dying at the same. I mourn and she whispers the story of renewal as if in apology, weathering my shadow so that in time I too can become a softer and more luminescent eye. Come and I might help shake loose from your soul your story, but as you love what is unveiled you might loathe it also, chancing to grasp your own shadow as the light falls around you. All I ask is that when your burdens become too much to bear you take your heart and deliver it to a source larger than yourself. By writing this (story) I invite the moon a little closer to home.

108

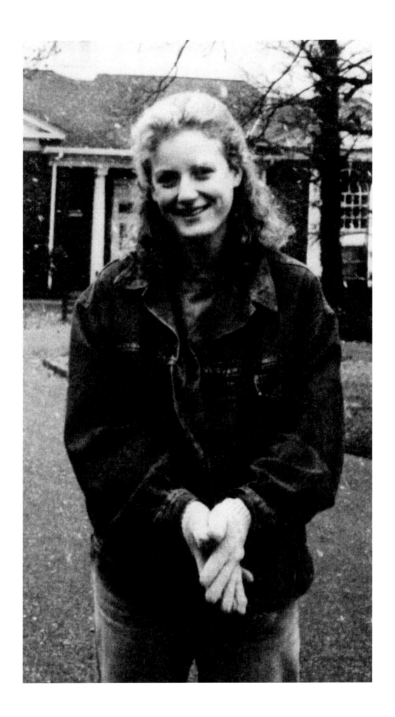

110